IT STARTED WITH HIPPOCRATES

The "Father of Medicine" was the first to note that substances which caused symptoms in well people often relieved those same symptoms in sick people. Many medical sages through the years added to these observations. Then, 200 years ago, Dr. Samuel Hahnemann codified this information and the results of his extensive researches into the art and science of homeopathy. Hahnemann's remarkable success in dealing with the devastating plagues of the era spread his therapy across Europe and eventually the world, and it now provides safe treatment which myriads of patients have found effective for a variety of conditions.

This concise guide to homeopathy details the nature of the treatment, types of remedies and how they are used, and provides an invaluable quick survey of homeopathic treatments for the most common injuries and ailments.

Trevor M. Cook, born in London, England, is known internationally for his work in the promotion and development of homeopathy. He is President of Dolisos Inc., a manufacturer of homeopathic medicines based in Las Vegas, Executive Director of the Society of Ultramolecular Medicine, editor of *American Homeopathy* and a member of the United States Pharmocopoeia Convention. He studied at the University of London.

Richard A. Passwater, Ph.D. is one of the most called-upon authorities for information relating to preventive health care. A noted biochemist, he is credited with popularizing the term "supernutrition," largely as a result of having written two bestsellers on the subject—*Supernutrition: Megavitamin Revolution* and *Supernutrition for Healthy Hearts.* His other books include *Easy No-Flab Diet, Cancer and Its Nutritional Therapies, Selenium as Food & Medicine, Trace Elements, Hair Analysis and Nutrition* (with Elmer M. Cranton, M.D.) and The Good Health Guide *The Antioxidants.*

Earl Mindell, R.Ph., Ph.D. combines the expertise and working experience of a pharmacist with extensive knowledge in most of the nutrition areas. *Earl Mindell's Vitamin Bible* is now a million-copy bestseller, and his more recent *Vitamin Bible for Your Kids* may very well duplicate his first *Bible*'s publishing history. His latest book is *Shaping Up with Vitamins.* Dr. Mindell's popular *Quick & Easy Guide to Better Health* is published by Keats Publishing, as is *The Vitamin Robbers,* a Good Health Guide.

A BEGINNER'S INTRODUCTION TO HOMEOPATHY

THE DRUGLESS ALTERNATE THERAPY THAT HAS HEALED MILLIONS

by Trevor M. Cook, Ph.D.

Keats Publishing, Inc. 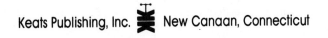 New Canaan, Connecticut

A Beginner's Introduction to Homeopathy is not intended as medical advice. Its intention is solely informational and educational. Please consult a medical or health professional should the need for one be indicated.

A BEGINNER'S INTRODUCTION TO HOMEOPATHY

Copyright © 1987 by Keats Publishing, Inc.

ISBN: 0-87983-394-7

Printed in the United States of America

Good Health Guides are published by
Keats Publishing, Inc.
27 Pine Street (Box 876)
New Canaan, Connecticut 06840

Contents

Homeopathy—a Real Alternative 1

What Is Homeopathy? 2

Is It a New Therapy? 3

What Are the Medicines Like? 6

Is Homeopathy Safe? 9

How Can I Receive Homeopathic Treatment? 10

Homeopathic Prescribing. 11

Homeopathic Treatment 13

Homeopathic Treatment of Common Ailments

   and First Aid 14

How Can the Remedies Be Obtained? 20

The Future of Homeopathy .21

Common Homeopathic Remedies 22

Bibliography 24

HOMEOPATHY—A REAL ALTERNATIVE

After the so-called miracle drug revolution, which began in the 1920s, won massive professional and public support, homeopathy with its comparatively mundane and unspectacular approach could not compete with the flood of drugs promising instant cures.

With growing concern over the side effects of modern synthetic drugs and drug addiction and the impersonal nature of conventional (allopathic) therapy, homeopathy is now staging a comeback worldwide.

Homeopathy is a safe, natural holistic therapy—a branch of medicine which views the patient and his or her illness in a fundamentally different way from modern allopathic medicine as practiced by most physicians.

WHAT IS HOMEOPATHY?

Homeopathy is a branch of medicine which views the patient and his or her illness in a fundamentally different way from the currently popular and now conventional allopathic approach. Homeopathic treatment itself is also different. Very small doses of natural drugs, which are completely safe, are prescribed.

The word "homeopathy" is derived from the Greek words *Homoios*, meaning similar or like, and *pathos*, meaning suffering. Hence, their combination means "like suffering," which embraces the basic principle of homeopathy, that is the treatment of like with like. That is, an illness is treated by selecting a remedy which has the ability to produce in a healthy person symptoms similar to those observed in the patient; the homeopathic remedy must be capable of producing in a healthy person suffering of a type similar to that experienced by the patient.

The "Law of Similars" may be more easily understood by comparison with conventional vaccination, which is closely analogous with homeopathy. Another example is the use of Belladonna (deadly nightshade) for the treatment of scarlet fever. The effects of Belladonna poisoning include flushed face, dilated pupils, high fever and a dry mouth. The symptoms of a flushed face and high fever are most prominent with a person suffering from scarlet fever; therefore, some doses of Belladonna may be prescribed for its treatment.

IS IT A NEW THERAPY?

Homeopathy is not an upstart therapy. It has been part of the entire fabric of medical practice for centuries. The principle of homeopathy was known even to the ancient Greeks. Hippocrates wrote of symptoms as the expression of nature's healing powers: "Through the like, disease is produced and through the application of the like, it is cured." The Swiss physician Paracelsus wrote in the 16th century that "sames must be cured by sames." Homeopathy sees the symptoms of a disease as the manifestation of the body's fight against that disease, that is, of its natural curative mechanism. The homeopathic physician, therefore, seeks to stimulate these symptoms rather than suppress them as in conventional medicine.

The founder of modern homeopathy is, however, generally acknowledged to be Samuel Hahnemann, who adopted the principle of homeopathy exclusively and developed it systematically. Born in Meissen in Saxony in 1755, he was a brilliant student and linguist and qualified in medicine at the University of Leipzig. He soon became a leading medical reformer and sought a more humane, compassionate and safer alternative to the barbaric and ineffective medical system which was then practiced.

Hahnemann discovered that small doses of the drug Cinchona, derived from the bark of a tree which contained a high level of quinine, could produce symptoms similar to malaria in a healthy person. He noted that, significantly, this drug had been used for some time for the effective treatment of malaria itself. He then conducted a series of systematic experiments with naturally-occurring remedies of animal, vegetable and mineral origin which produced symptoms similar to a wide range of diseases, thus establishing the "like with like" principle. These experiments he called "provings," and this approach continues to be the fundamental method for the discovery of new homeopathic medicines.

Having established the basic principle of homeopathy, Hahnemann proceeded to determine the smallest effective doses in order to make the treatment as safe as possible. He produced what he termed "potencies" by the serial dilution of alcoholic extracts of the individual drugs, followed by a process known as "succussion," that is, vigorous shaking with impact. These potencies are therefore a measure of the relative dilution of the concentrated drug and they are denoted by a number which follows the name of the drug itself. For example, Arnica 6x or Sulfur 30x: the higher the number the greater the dilution. These minute quantities—even the 6th (centesimal) potency is a dilution of one part of the drug in 1 trillion parts of the diluent—render the substance completely safe. The curative properties of even highly toxic substances are released at these extremely high dilutions.

Today, there are over 2,000 homeopathic remedies normally prescribed in potencies ranging from 3x (or 1/1000 dilution, prepared by three 1/10 dilutions with succussion) to 12c (an extremely dilute solution prepared by twelve 1/100 dilutions with succussion) capable of treating a wide range of acute and chronic diseases safely and effectively.

Another important feature of homeopathy is that illness is not considered to be localized, but to involve the whole person, both physically and psychologically, within his or her total environment. It is, therefore, a highly personalized treatment and is truly a "holistic" medicine. Homeopathy concentrates on treating the whole patient rather than the disease. The homeopathic doctor is concerned not only with the symptoms exhibited by the patient, but with the patient's physical appearance, his or her likes and dislikes and temperament. Patients suffering from the same disease may often be treated with different remedies because people are different.

Subsequently, Samuel Hahnemann demonstrated the effectiveness of homeopathy in the treatment of a serious epidemic of typhoid following the Battle of Leipzig in 1813 and of cholera, which scourged Europe in the winter of 1831–2. At his death in 1843, homeopathic treatment was common in over 60 countries throughout the world; in many countries it was the preferred therapy. In America at the turn of the century there were 25 homeopathic medical colleges and hospitals.

The decline of homeopathy in the early 20th century is a matter of history—no doubt hastened by the so-called "miracle drug" revolution in the 30s and 40s. But today homeopathy is enjoying an astonishing growth of interest and support in America. Many factors may have influenced this trend, including fear of side effects of conventional drugs and the desire to be treated as a person and not simply a bearer of disease.

WHAT ARE THE MEDICINES LIKE?

Homeopathic medicines look exactly like any other medicine, although their mode of action is quite different. They are taken the same way as conventional medicines, in the form of tablets, granules, liquids or ointments. The solid forms are all sweet-tasting since they are prepared from pure forms of sugar (sucrose or 20 percent sucrose in a lactose base).

Sources of the Medicines

The medicines are not synthetic, as are conventional medicines, and are all derived from natural sources—vegetable, animal and mineral. Over 60 percent of all homeopathic medicines—more than 2,000 of them—are prepared from vegetable or plant materials, including flowers, vegetables, shrubs, the bark of trees, roots, berries, fruits, buds or young shoots, seeds and bulbs or corms. Some examples:

Atropa Belladonna (Deadly nightshade)—prepared from the whole plant at the commencement of flowering.
Calendula Officinalis (Common marigold)—prepared from the top section of the fresh flowering plant.
Cinchona (Peruvian bark, Quinaquina tree)—prepared from the bark of the tree.

Many homeopathic medicines are prepared from naturally-occurring mineral substances, including metals, non-metallic substances and mineral salts, for example:

Kalium Bichromicum (Potassium dichromate)—from chromium iron ore.

Calcarea Carbonica (Calcium carbonate)—extracted from the middle layer of the oyster shell.

Graphites (Pure carbon)—black lead such as found in the lead of a pencil.

Animal sources of homeopathic medicines are most varied and exotic, and form a very important group. Among them are:

Sepia—the "ink" or juice of the cuttlefish.

Lachesis mutus (Bushmaster snake)—the poisonous venom of the snake.

Apis Mellifera—the whole honeybee.

Preparation of the Medicines

The first stage in the preparation of all the medicines is to produce the medicine in its most concentrated form, which is called the mother tincture. Plant or animal materials are macerated; minerals are ground to a fine powder and extracted with pure alcohol. The resulting suspension is filtered to produce the mother tincture as a clear although often yellowish or brownish liquid.

Substances which are insoluble in alcohol are ground to form an intimate mixture with pure lactose. This process is known as trituration and produces a solid mother tincture.

The procedure developed by Hahnemann for the dilution of these mother tinctures to produce the decimal series or the centesimal series of potencies has been previously described. Homeopathic preparations are not simple dilutions, but are prepared by a rigid procedure involving both serial dilution and succussion. The final stage of the preparation of the medicines involves the impregnation of pure lactose or lactose-sucrose granules or tablets with the liquid potencies.

Care of the Medicines

Homeopathic medicines are very sensitive, and as they

contain infinitesimally small amounts of the active ingredient, they can easily become contaminated. They are best stored in glass (not plastic) containers, and tablets or granules should not be touched with the hand. Use the cap to hold them and drop directly into the mouth.

Store the medicines in a cool, dark place away from strong smells, such as garlic or camphor. Keep the containers well stoppered. Properly stored, they should retain their potency for at least five years.

IS HOMEOPATHY SAFE?

By virtue of the very, very small doses employed in homeopathic treatment, the medicines are completely safe. Although a slight aggravation of symptoms may be experienced, as a result of the "like with like" principle being called into practice, these are no unwanted side effects. Where dosing instructions have been followed, no case of any toxic action has ever been reported associated with homeopathic medicines.

Furthermore, homeopathic medicines, unlike many conventional drugs, are nonaddictive and are completely safe, even for babies and children.

Since the medicines are not quantitative in their action, it is not dangerous if the prescribed dose is exceeded in error.

HOW CAN I RECEIVE HOMEOPATHIC TREATMENT?

Although homeopathy is not taught at the major medical schools in America, it is practiced mainly by regular, fully qualified M.D.s who have studied homeopathy in post-graduate courses. Lists of homeopathic physicians may be obtained from various homeopathic organizations.

As homeopathy is holistic—that is, a therapy which involves the whole person—many acupuncturists, chiropractors and naturopaths who have adopted a holistic approach have included homeopathy in their treatment programs.

Since homeopathic medicines are quite safe, they are suitable for self-help or first-aid treatment in the home. They are available to the public in some regular pharmacies and even health food stores. They may be purchased over the counter without a prescription. These medicines are sold in lower potencies only or they are sold as combinations of several remedies as "specialties," with a specific indication for their use on the label, for example, tablets for the treatment of colds or granules for the treatment of indigestion.

HOMEPATHIC PRESCRIBING

As an holistic therapy, the prescribing of homeopathic medicines is necessarily concerned with the symptoms, the drug and the person.

In establishing the diagnosis and treatment appropriate for that diagnosis in a particular patient, both signs (that is, objective evidence perceptible to the examiner) and symptoms (that is, subjective evidence such as pain perceived and described by the patient) must be considered.

It is then necessary to identify certain salient characteristics in the patient's personality or constitution. These characteristics may be physical, such as whether the patient has dark hair or fair hair, whether the patient is fat or thin, tall or short, or has a dry skin or a moist skin. The mental characteristics must also be taken into account. Whether the patient is gregarious or prefers to be alone, whether practical or artistically inclined, and the patient's likes and dislikes, will affect treatment.

Factors that make the condition better (ameliorations) or worse (aggravations), called the modalities, must also be considered. These include thermal modalities (better or worse for hot or cold), time modalities (better or worse at different times of the day) and physical modalities—better or worse for exercise or rest, standing up or lying down, etc.).

Homeopathic remedies may be classified as follows:

Polycrest Remedies

These remedies, named "polycrest" by Samuel Hahnemann, are effective for a wide range of symptoms and conditions. The personality element is minimal, and they are equally suitable for most types of people. Examples of polycrest remedies are Arnica, Nux Vomica, Ignatia, Graphites, Silica and Sulfur.

Constitutional Remedies

Remedies which are effective for most conditions of specific types of people. These are "person-oriented" remedies, for example the "Pulsatilla type" or the "Sepia type." In general, constitutional remedies are used for chronic or recurring diseases.

Specific Remedies

Specific remedies are the opposite of constitutional remedies in that they may be prescribed for a specific ailment for all types of patient personalities. These remedies may be described as "symptom-oriented" rather than "person-oriented." Thus, for example, we have Thuja Occidentalis, which is almost a specific for warts, and Colchicum Autumnale, a near specific for the treatment of gout.

Combination Remedies

Single homeopathic remedies may be combined effectively by a skilled homeopathic physician to cover the totality of symptoms. This technique is sometimes called polypharmacy.

Increasing use is being made of combinations of up to eight single remedies. For common conditions, such as coughs, sore throat, acne, or hay fever, combination therapy has been shown to be most effective. If the elements of the combination are carefully selected not to offset or interfere with one another, the combined effect may be synergistic.

HOMEOPATHIC TREATMENT

Homeopathic medicines are prescribed for most common and serious conditions, both acute and chronic. In general, frequent doses are employed at lower potencies for acute conditions of short duration, whereas less frequent doses—one dose per day, or even one dose per week—at higher potencies are employed for chronic conditions. The frequency of the dose depends entirely on the severity of the symptoms.

Lower potencies commonly prescribed are 6x and 12x, and higher potencies commonly prescribed are 200c or 1M (1000c).

The standard dosage for all homeopathic medicines is 5 granules for an adult or 3 granules for a child, dissolved under the tongue. For liquid medicines, the standard dosage is 10 drops on the tongue. When they are taken, the mouth should be clean and free of strong-smelling substances. The doses are most effective when taken between meals or at least two hours before meals. Coffee, tea and alcohol should be avoided during homeopathic treatment.

As with any other medical treatment, regular exercise, adequate rest and proper diet are recommended to aid recovery.

Dosing should be continued until improvement is evident, at which time the interval between doses may be increased. When the condition is cleared, the dosing should be discontinued. The dosing should be repeated only if the original symptoms recur.

HOMEOPATHIC TREATMENT OF COMMON AILMENTS AND FIRST AID

Self-treatment with homeopathic medicines is relatively simple. Most common, day-to-day ailments experienced by almost everyone respond well to homeopathic treatment. These ailments are mainly acute conditions, with a rapid onset of symptoms which persist only for relatively short periods. As previously explained, such conditions respond most effectively to treatment by homeopathic medicines in low potencies, such as 6x or 12x potency.

For more serious conditions a qualified physician should be consulted.

Accidents and Injuries

For mental and physical shock, fright with palpitations, gasping for breath, collapse or distress take Aconite. This remedy is particularly useful immediately following a shock or involvement in an accident, even the shock arising as a result of witnessing an accident.

Arnica may be used to reduce the prolonged effects of a shock or injury. This remedy is particularly effective in the treatment of bruises and contusions where the skin is unbroken. Pain and swelling after a dental extraction, sprains of joints, or fractured bones may all be relieved with the internal administration of Arnica.

For collapse or fainting Carbo Vegetabilis is the preferred remedy, particularly when the patient is cold.

Painful injuries to the nerves, as in crushed fingertips or toes, animal bites or penetrating puncture wounds, such as treading on a nail, respond to treatment with Hypericum. Arnica may be taken immediately after the injury.

Burns

Where painful blisters result which burn when touched, Cantharus should be taken for relief. Cantharus should also be used for burns of the chest and face. In less severe burns, Urtica Urens may be applied as a lotion and taken internally to relieve the pain.

Headache

Belladonna is recommended for the throbbing headache, particularly if accompanied with a red, flushed face. Headaches that respond well to homeopathic treatment with Belladonna usually come on suddenly and may be worse in the afternoon or at night. Belladonna will be particularly effective for lively individuals who may be subject to temper.

However, if the pain is lessened when the head is bent backwards, Hypericum may be the answer. If it is right-sided and worse for movement of the head, then the remedy of choice is Bryonia, which may also be used if the headache occurs in association with respiratory infection or cough which aggravates the pain.

Headaches resulting from mental exertion, excitement or overwork may be treated with Argentum Nitricum. Such headaches may have a gradual onset and there may be tenseness or stiffness around the neck. The pain spreads over to the left temple and the head may be tender to touch.

One homeopathic remedy, Lachesis, is particularly helpful for headaches occuring during the menopause and when it is worse on waking in the morning.

Finally, the hangover-type headache, following overindulgence in eating and drinking with the "morning after" feeling. This is usually cleared by Nux Vomica. The Nux Vomica type of individual is slim, dark-haired and inclined to be impatient or irritable.

Colds

If the cold comes on suddenly or after exposure to drafts or cold winds, the remedy is Aconite. When the eyes are streaming and there is an acrid discharge from the nose, sneezing and headache, then the remedy which may be most effective is Allium Cepa. In these cases, the patient may be hot and thirsty and feel better in the open air.

When the cold symptoms are influenza-like, with possibly a headache, the remedy is Gelsemium.

Colds with much nasal discharge, when the nose is "running like a tap," and lachrymation with violent sneezing are best treated by Natrium Muriaticum. There may be severe headaches and the sufferer feels worse for heat, but better from cold.

Sore Throat

Sudden onset of a sore throat with red, flushed face and red tongue and dilated pupils is best treated by Belladonna.

If there is an offensive discharge and profuse sweating associated with a sore throat, the remedy of choice is Hepar Sulfuris.

Sore throat beginning on the left side and moving to the right side suggests using Lachesis. In these cases the throat is extremely sensitive to touch and worse from hot drink. There may also be a dislike of any constriction around the neck and there may be a marked aggravation after sleep.

A right-sided sore throat which is improved by warm drinks may be treeated with Lycopodium. Intense, conscientious people may find Lycopodium particularly beneficial.

Boils and Abscesses

If they are inflamed and very sensitive, better with heat and worse from pressure, Hepar Sulfuris is recommended. Recurring spots associated with skin eruptions, heat and itching may be treated with Sulfur. The Sulfur patient may tend to sweat easily and have a nervous yet independent nature.

Rheumatism

The most commonly used remedy for rheumatism is Rhus Toxicodendron (poison ivy). It is characterized by burning pains and stiffness in any part of the body in muscles, tendons and joints. An important modality is that pain is worse on first moving but is relieved on continued movement. The pain is better for heat but worse at night.

If the rheumatic pains are burning and shooting like electric shocks, then the remedy to chose is Phytolacca. These pains may be worse on motion or during the night or in damp weather.

In contrast to Rhus Toxicodendron, if the symptoms are worse for movement, then the remedy is Bryonia. Other symptoms in this case may be a dry tongue and a great thirst with despair or despondency.

If the rheumatic pains move from joint to joint and are very sensitive to touch, then Colchicum Autumnale may prove effective. This remedy is widely used for the treatment of gout. The pain is worse in cold, damp weather, especially in the autumn and winter.

Rheumatic pain in the legs and knees with stiffness and weariness may be relieved by Berberis.

Chilblains

If the chilblains are bright red with some swelling, then Belladonna may be taken, but if they are bright red and inflamed with burning, itching and blistering, Rhus Toxicodendron is recommended. In most cases, Tamus ointment may be applied externally.

Coughs

The dry cough with a painful chest which is worse on lying down and at night may be treated effectively with Bryonia. A dry cough with hoarseness which is worse on talking is better treated with Phosphorus.

A cough producing yellow, stringy sputum may be treated by Kalium Bichromicum.

The short, dry, irritating cough which is always worse at night is treated with Aconite.

Catarrh

Yellow, stringy catarrh with sore throat and hoarseness may be treated with Kalium Bichromicum. These symptoms will invariably be worse in the morning. If the catarrh is thick and yellow-green in color, often associated with a head cold, then Calcarea Fluorica is preferred. These symptoms may be worse after rest.

Chilly individuals suffering from catarrh, who may have an unhealthy complexion and constipation, will find treatment with Natrium Muriaticum effective.

Watering eyes and a running nose, with the catarrh worse in the evening and in bed, suggest the use of Euphrasia.

Gout

Colchicum Autumnale, the Autumn Crocus, is almost a specific and is useful for most cases of gout. Such cases may be accompanied by weakness or nausea and swelling of the big toe. All these symptoms may be worse for movement.

In the early stages of gout, Pulsatilla may be taken.

Diarrhea

Proper diet is always recommended for diarrhea. These are a few homeopathic remedies that will help different types of diarrhea.

If there is restlessness with vomiting arising from mild food poisoning and there are frequent, dark stools, then Arsenicum Album is recommended. Diarrhea resulting from overeating or from eating artificial foods, and with passing only a small quantity with each attempt, is best treated with Nux Vomica. Treatment with Nux Vomica of infants with diarrhea is particularly effective.

If the stools are greenish-white and slimy and the patient is also suffering from stomachache, the remedy may be Chamomilla. This remedy is most effective with teething infants.

Bites and Stings

Immediately following an insect sting, such as a bee or wasp sting, take Apis Mellifera. Such stings may be red and swollen and this strongly indicates Apis Mellifera. A useful substitute for the treatment of bee or other insect stings is Urtica Urens.

HOW CAN THE REMEDIES BE OBTAINED?

Homeopathic medicines will, of course, be prescribed by qualified homeopathic physicians. Homeopathy is also practiced by other therapists, such as chiropractors, acupuncturists or naturopaths who regard homeopathy as complementary to their own form of medical treatment.

Because homeopathic medicines are intrinsically safe, they may be purchased over the counter at an increasing number of regular pharmacies and some health food stores.

Homeopathic medicines are particularly suited to self-help and first-aid treatment and many people find it desirable to keep a "first-aid kit" of the remedies at home. These remedies for simple ailments may be purchased directly from the manufacturers.

THE FUTURE OF HOMEOPATHY

Homeopathy today is gaining more support than at any time since early this century. This trend will continue as more and more physicians practice homeopathy and more and more people receive homeopathic treatment. Since the death of Samuel Hahnemann, homeopathy has been interwoven with the entire fabric of modern medical practice, and this fact will inevitably become generally recognized.

Homeopathy will not, however, be totally accepted by the medical establishment until it becomes part of the undergraduate syllabus at medical schools. Further legislation will also be required in most countries in Europe and in America to confirm the acceptance of homeopathy and clearly define the rights of those physicians who wish to practice it.

The ultimate key to its acceptance is, like any other field of medicine, to show undeniable evidence of its effectiveness. Homeopathy must also be dynamic and flexible and in a continual state of evolution. These objectives may only be achieved through further research. Since 1950, scientific experimentation has supplemented clinical experience and research workers have striven to show the validity of fundamental homeopathic principles.

Whole new branches of homeopathy have been opened up. The main new branch is known as the biotherapies, which include:

Organotherapy—dilutions of organs, glands and tissues
Gemmotherapy—dilutions of buds or young shoots of
plants

Lithotherapy—dilutions of natural minerals or rocks
Isotherapy—dilutions of the agent responsible for an illness (taken from the patient)

The immense potential of homeopathy is demonstrated when we consider that about 2,000 of the existing remedies are derived from plant sources, yet there are over half a million plant species on earth.

COMMON HOMEOPATHIC REMEDIES

Full Name	*Abbreviated Name*
Aconitum Napellus	Aconite
Actaea Racemosa	Actaea Rac.
Apis Mellifera	Apis Mel.
Argentum Nitricum	Argentum Nit.
Arnica Montana	Arnica
Arsenicum Album	Arsen. Alb.
Atropa Belladonna	Belladonna
Berberis Vulgaris	Berberis
Bryonia Alba	Bryonia
Calcarea Carbonica	Calc. Carb.
Calcarea Fluorica	Calc. Fluor.
Calcarea Phosphorica	Calc. Phos.
Calendula Officinalis	Calendula
Cantharis Vesicatoria	Cantharis
Carbo Vegetabilis	Carbo Veg.
Chamomilla	Chamomilla
Chelidonium Majus	Chelidonium
Cocculus Indicus	Cocculus

Full Name	Abbreviated Name
Colchicum Autumnale	Colchicum
Cuprum Metallicum	Cuprum Met.
Drosera Rotundifolia	Drosera
Euphrasia Officinalis	Euphrasia
Ferrum Phosphoricum	Ferrum Phos.
Graphites	Graphites
Hamamelis Virginiana	Hamamelis
Hepar Sulfuris	Hepar Sulf.
Hydrastis Canadensis	Hydrastis
Hypericum Perforatum	Hypericum
Ignatia Amara	Ignatia
Ipecacuanha	Ipecacuanha
Kalium Bichromicum	Kali Bich.
Kalium Phosphoricum	Kali Phos.
Lachesis Mutus	Lachesis
Lycopodium Clavatum	Lycopodium
Magnesia Phosphorica	Mag. Phos.
Mercurius Vivus	Merc. Viv.
Natrium Muriaticum	Natrium Mur.
Nux Vomica	Nux Vomica
Phosphorus	Phosphorus
Phytolacca Decandra	Phytolacca
Pulsatilla Nigricans	Pulsatilla
Rhus Toxicodendron	Rhus Tox.
Ruta Graveolens	Ruta Grav.
Sepia Officinalis	Sepia
Silica	Silica
Sulfur	Sulfur
Symphytum Officinale	Symphytum
Thuja Occidentalis	Thuja
Urtica Urens	Urtica Urens
Veratrum Album	Veratrum Alb.

BIBLIOGRAPHY

Borland, D. M. *Homeopathy in Practice*. New Canaan, Conn.: Keats Publishing, 1983.

Boyd, H. *Introduction to Homeopathic Medicine*. New Canaan, Conn.: Keats Publishing, 1983.

Clarke, J. H. *The Prescriber*. Hengiscote, Devon, UK: Health Science Press, 1972.

Cook, T. M. *The A–Z of Homeopathy*. Slough, Berks., UK: Foulsham, 1985.

———, *Samuel Hahnemann—Founder of Homeopathic Medicine*. Wellingborough , Northants, UK: Thorsons Publishers, 1984.

Hamlyn, E. C. *The Healing Art of Homeopathy*. New Canaan, Conn.: Keats Publishing, 1979.

Julian, O. A. *Materia Medica of New Homeopathic Remedies*. New Canaan, Conn.: Keats Publishing, 1979.

Pratt, N. J. *Homeopathic Prescribing*. New Canaan, Conn.: Keats Publishing, 1983.

Smith, T. *Homeopathic Medicine*. Wellingborough, Northants., UK: Thorsons Publishers, 1982.

Now that you have been introduced to Homeopathy —

Here are six ways to get the whole inspiring story of an age-old, yet new, force in medicine, and how it can help assure your better health!

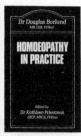

HOMEOPATHY IN PRACTICE
Douglas Borland, M.D.
Paperback $9.95
The author covers a variety of complaints and disorders, offers detailed guidance on their treatment by homeopathy.

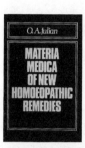

MATERIA MEDICA OF NEW HOMEOPATHIC REMEDIES
O.A. Julian, M.D.
Paperback $29.95
Back in print! Over 100 new remedies in a 626-page book which includes a repertory of symptoms and an index.

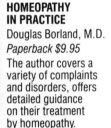

HOMEOPATHIC PRESCRIBING
Noel Pratt, M.D.
Paperback $8.95
One hundred and fifty-nine common complaints are covered, arranged alphabetically for easy reference.

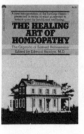

THE HEALING ART OF HOMEOPATHY
Edward Hamlyn, M.D.
Paperback $5.95
A new interpretation of Hahnemann's ORGANON in which the essentials of this new force in medicine are described.

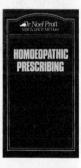

INTRODUCTION TO HOMEOPATHIC MEDICINE
Hamish Boyd, M.D.
Paperback $14.95
A book for practitioners with practical information on homeopathic caretaking and diagnosis and the application of remedies.

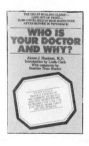

WHO IS YOUR DOCTOR AND WHY?
Alonzo Shadman, M.D.
Paperback $3.95
Includes the famous 190-page "Pointers to the Common Remedies" — hundreds of ailments and the homeopathic remedies to use for home first aid.

In case your local book store or health store does not have it — use this page (and next) as an order form/envelope to order the copies you need direct from the publisher.

Order Form

Please rush me the following books in quantities indicated:

___ copies **Homeopathy in Practice** $9.95
___ copies **Homeopathic Prescribing** $8.95
___ copies **Intro. Homeopathic Medicine** $14.95
___ copies **Materia Medica** $29.95
___ copies **Healing Art of Homeopathy** $5.95
___ copies **Who Is Your Doctor and Why?** $3.95

I enclose $ _____ plus $2.00 postage & handling   TOTAL $ _____

OR charge my _ Visa _ MasterCard Acct. #_____ Expires _ / _ / _

Your signature (if charged) _____

Your name _____ Address _____

City _____ State _____ Zip _____

At your favorite book store or health store or use this page to order direct from the publisher. Please scotch tape — do not staple. Check or money order, please. No cash.

- -

From _____

_____

_____

Place
Stamp
Here

TO
Keats Publishing, Inc.
27 Pine Street (Box 876)
New Canaan, CT 06840

Att'n Mail Order Department